Gynecologic and Obstetric Prophylactic Hemostasis by Intra-arterial Balloon Occlusion

Satoru Takeda • Ryohei Kuwatsuru
Editors

Gynecologic and Obstetric Prophylactic Hemostasis by Intra-arterial Balloon Occlusion

Springer

Editors
Satoru Takeda
Department of Obstetrics and Gynecology
Juntendo University Faculty of Medicine
Tokyo
Japan

Ryohei Kuwatsuru
Department of Radiology
Juntendo University Faculty of Medicine
Tokyo
Japan

ISBN 978-981-10-8832-2   ISBN 978-981-10-8833-9 (eBook)
https://doi.org/10.1007/978-981-10-8833-9

Library of Congress Control Number: 2018948849

Printed on acid-free paper

This Springer imprint is published by the registered company Springer Nature Singapore Pte Ltd.
The registered company address is: 152 Beach Road, #21-01/04 Gateway East, Singapore 189721, Singapore

Preface

Obstetricians have long had to contend with bleeding during delivery and cesarean section and gynecologists have faced similar challenges during tumor resection. Even today, bleeding is a major cause of death in pregnant women. Thirty-odd years ago, when I was a resident, I performed a hysterectomy on a woman with a low-lying placenta and a history of cesarean section. Hysterectomy was required because bleeding from the uterine surface of the detached placenta was uncontrollable. The bleeding volume was 7000 mL. This was the first case of placenta accreta I experienced. After 7 years of training in a university hospital, I set out for my new position at a hospital that became the first general perinatal center in Japan. Several years later, we treated two pregnant women with a history of cesarean section who had massive bleeding during repeat cesarean and were transferred from other hospitals. One case was dead on arrival, and the other underwent repeat laparotomy, partial cystectomy, and hysterectomy. Despite disseminated intravascular coagulation, and a bleeding volume well over 20,000 mL, the patient was saved. Contending with bleeding is an ongoing problem.

Throughout history, warfare has necessitated the development of innovative medical technologies and new treatments. In the Korean War, hemostatic "intra-aortic balloon catheter tamponade" (Hughes CW. Surgery. 1954;36:65–8) was actually used to control abdominal bleeding due to trauma, and cases were subsequently reported in the literature. Thereafter, temporary hemostasis using an intra-arterial balloon catheter was introduced in trauma management and is now widely used for resuscitative endovascular balloon occlusion of the aorta in emergency medicine. Use of this technique has been extended for prevention of massive bleeding during hysterectomy in cases of placenta previa accreta.

Interventional radiology has made remarkable advances, and hemostasis using transcatheter arterial embolization or temporary intra-arterial balloon occlusion is now widely performed. These techniques have enabled minimally invasive hemostasis without the use of surgical procedures, contributing to the saving of lives. In this book, specialists in radiology, obstetrics, and gynecology describe current techniques of prophylactic hemostasis in the field of obstetrics and gynecology. I hope that physicians will read between the lines and appreciate the efforts of those who have contended with bleeding for many years.

I invite clinicians to embrace this book as a guide to the avoidance of massive bleeding and the need for blood transfusions as a means of improving patient care.

Tokyo, Japan Satoru Takeda
Tokyo, Japan Ryohei Kuwatsuru
January 2018

Contents

Anatomy of Uterine Blood Supply and the Prevention of Massive Hemorrhage

1

Hitomi Kato and Ryohei Kuwatsuru

Abstract

Embolization of uterine artery is sometimes required to prevent the massive hemorrhage after the delivery. Knowledge of uterine artery anatomy makes catheterization easy. In this chapter, four anatomical types of uterine artery are described with the angiographic images as well as the ovarian artery anatomy.

Keywords

Uterine artery · Ovarian artery · Anatomy

1.1 Introduction

When treating the uterine vasculature, it is vital to correctly select the target vessels, such as the uterine arteries. Because the arteries of the pelvis follow a complex course and the internal iliac artery has many branches apart from the uterine arteries, including both parietal and visceral branches, knowledge of the vascular anatomy of this region is important.

1.2 Anatomy

The abdominal aorta bifurcates into the left and right common iliac arteries, often at a level between the middle 1/3 of the fourth lumbar vertebrae and the upper 1/3 of the fifth lumbar vertebrae [1]. Each common iliac artery bifurcates into an internal

H. Kato (✉) · R. Kuwatsuru
Department of Radiology, Juntendo University Faculty of Medicine, Tokyo, Japan
e-mail: hikatou@juntendo.ac.jp

S. Takeda, R. Kuwatsuru (eds.), *Gynecologic and Obstetric Prophylactic Hemostasis by Intra-arterial Balloon Occlusion*, https://doi.org/10.1007/978-981-10-8833-9_1

iliac artery and external iliac artery anterior to the sacroiliac articulation, and the internal iliac artery then branches into anterior and posterior divisions. The anterior division gives off both visceral and parietal branches, whereas the posterior gives rise only to parietal branches.

The median sacral artery arises from the posterior surface of the abdominal aorta superior to its bifurcation and descends in front of the vertebral bodies.

Eighty-one percent to 91% of ovarian arteries arise from the abdominal aorta (Fig. 1.1). Seventy percent of gonadal arteries arise from the ventral surface of the abdominal aorta a few centimeters below the origin of the renal arteries. However, up to 20% of gonadal arteries originate from the renal arteries [2].

The internal iliac artery has parietal branches and visceral branches.

The parietal branches are the iliolumbar artery, lateral sacral artery, obturator artery, superior gluteal artery, and inferior gluteal artery. The visceral branches are the uterine artery, superior vesical artery, inferior vesical artery (the vaginal artery in females), middle rectal artery, and internal pudendal artery.

A rare congenital anomaly is the existence of a persistent sciatic artery as a communication of the internal iliac artery into the thigh.

The key to performing uterine artery embolization successfully is a profound understanding of the anatomy of the uterine artery.

Gomez et al. classified the patterns of the uterine artery as types I–IV [2, 3].

Type I: Uterine artery is the first branch of the inferior gluteal artery (45%) (Fig. 1.2).

Type II: Uterine artery is the second or third branch of the inferior gluteal artery (6%) (Fig. 1.3).

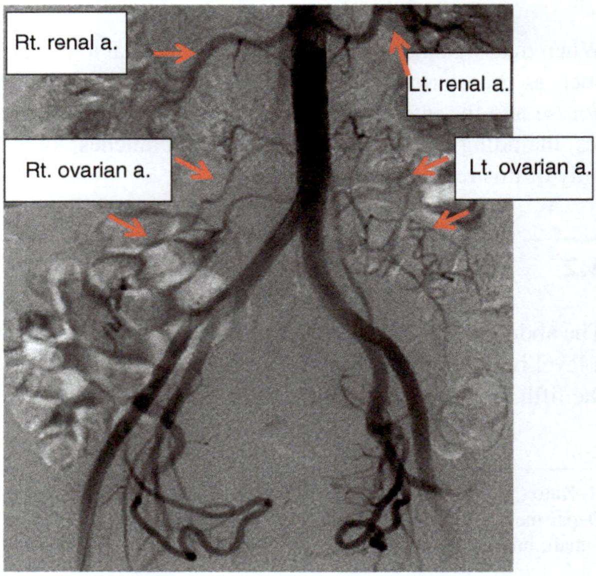

Fig. 1.1 Ovarian arteries

Fig. 1.2 Type I uterine artery (oblique view)

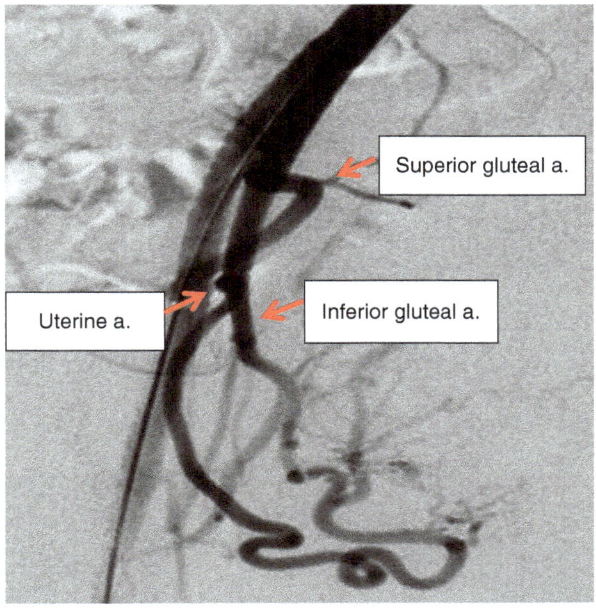

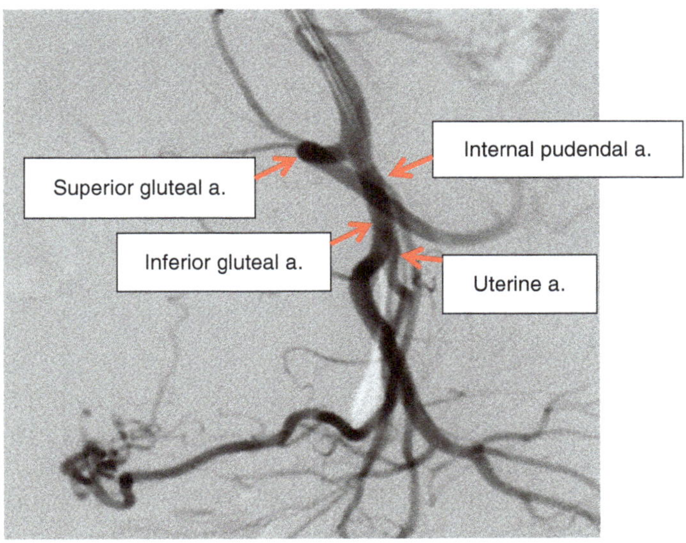

Fig. 1.3 Type II uterine artery (oblique view)

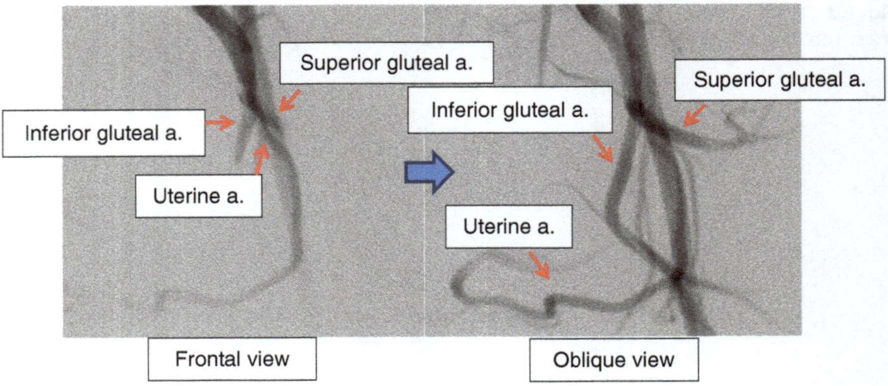

Fig. 1.4 Type III uterine artery (frontal and oblique view)

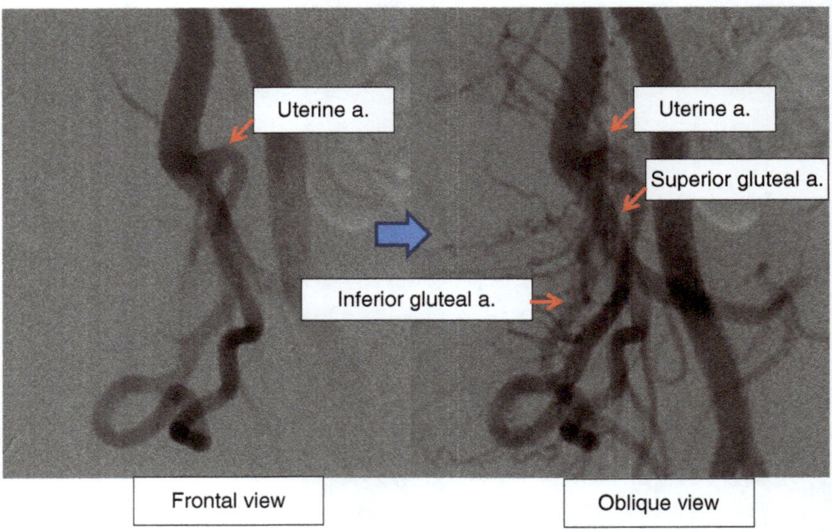

Fig. 1.5 Type IV uterine artery (frontal and oblique view)

Type III: Uterine artery, inferior gluteal artery, and superior gluteal artery branch off at the same level (trifurcation) (43%) (Fig. 1.4).

Type IV: Uterine artery is the first branch of the internal iliac artery (above the level of the inferior gluteal and superior gluteal arteries) (6%) (Fig. 1.5).

Each uterine artery has several branches. The uterine artery diverges anteriorly from the internal iliac artery and bifurcates into descending and ascending branches. The ascending branch anastomoses with the ovarian arcade to form an arterial arcade.

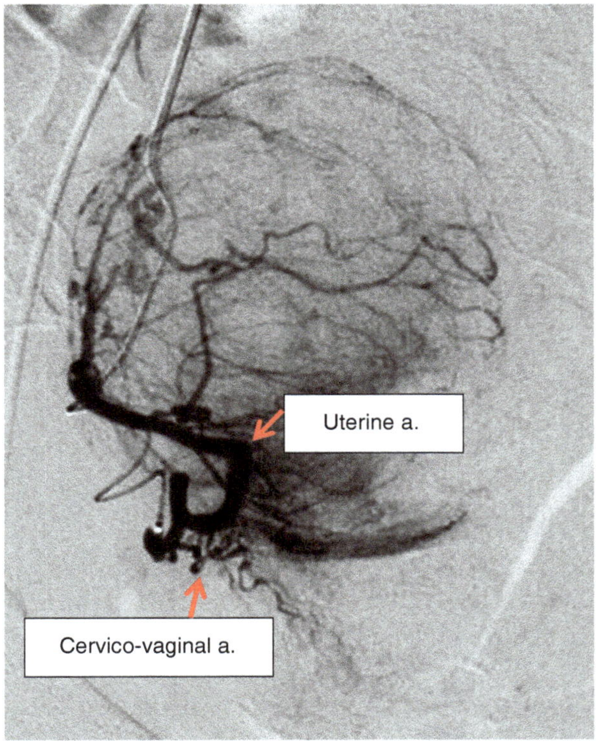

Fig. 1.6 Cervicovaginal artery

The superior vesical artery arises from the internal iliac artery near the origin of the uterine artery and courses roughly parallel to the descending uterine artery.

The cervicovaginal artery diverges from the arcade artery of the uterine artery (Fig. 1.6).

1.3 Prophylaxis of Bleeding by Uterine Artery Embolization

Prophylactic uterine artery embolization in the obstetrics domain is applied on a case-by-case basis when massive hemorrhage is expected at the time of surgeries such as cesarean section or hysterectomy for placenta accreta or placenta previa. In these cases, arterial balloon occlusion may be performed before surgery, or uterine artery embolization may be performed after delivery. Arteries occluded by the balloon may include the abdominal aorta, both common iliac arteries, or both internal iliac arteries. After delivery, multiple embolic agents, such as gelatin sponges, coils, or N-butyl cyanoacrylate (NBCA)–lipiodol, are used for uterine artery embolization, because the blood flow in the uterine artery differs among patients and is sometimes copious.

References

1. Anson BJ, et al. The topographical positions and the mutual relations of the visceral branches of the abdominal aorta. Anat Rec. 1936;67:7–15.
2. Gomez-Jorge J. Pelvic anatomy relevant in uterine embolization. In: Spies JB, Pelage JP, editors. Uterine artery embolization and gynecologic embolotherapy. Philadelphia: Lippincott Williams and Wilkins; 2004. p. 19–27.
3. Gomez-Jorge J, et al. Uterine artery anatomy relevant to uterine leiomyomata embolization. Cardiovasc Intervent Radiol. 2003;26:522–7.

Application and Methods of the Arterial Balloon Occlusion for the Prophylaxis of Massive Hemorrhage in Gynecologic Fields

2

Akihiko Shiraishi

Abstract
We reveal the endovascular technique of the perioperative placement of arterial occlusion balloons catheters at the internal iliac arteries in reducing intraoperative blood loss for the prophylaxis of massive hemorrhage in gynecologic fields.

Keywords
Massive hemorrhage · Prophylaxis · Balloon occlusion · Internal iliac artery

All balloon occlusion catheters are placed by the interventional radiologist in the angiography suite. First, bilateral femoral arterial puncture is performed by using 5- or 6-French vascular sheaths under local anesthesia. The vascular anatomy then is evaluated through pelvic aortography using a 4-French pigtail catheter, after which a 5.5-French cobra catheter (Selecon MP Catheter II; Terumo Clinical Supply, Gifu, Japan) over a 0.035-in. angled guidewire is used under fluoroscopic guidance to cannulate the contralateral internal iliac artery. By passing the catheter through crossover sheaths in the contralateral common femoral artery, the tip of the balloon catheter is positioned in the proximal portion of the internal iliac artery, past the bifurcation of the common iliac artery. A test volume of dilute water-soluble contrast material is injected to inflate the occlusion balloons to the optimal size. Care is

A. Shiraishi
Department of Radiology, Juntendo University, Faculty of Medicine, Tokyo, Japan
e-mail: asiraisi@juntendo.ac.jp

S. Takeda, R. Kuwatsuru (eds.), *Gynecologic and Obstetric Prophylactic Hemostasis by Intra-arterial Balloon Occlusion*, https://doi.org/10.1007/978-981-10-8833-9_2

taken in determining the volume required, because overinflation of compliant balloons may result in arterial rupture. A 50:50 contrast/saline solution then is used for test inflations sufficient to occlude the internal iliac artery, which is verified through injection of contrast via the catheter lumen followed by digital subtraction angiography. The volume needed to assure arterial occlusion is usually less than 0.4 mL, and the same volume is subsequently used to inflate the balloons during the surgery itself. All sheaths and balloon catheters are covered with tape. After the procedure, the patient is transported from the intervention room to the operating room. The balloon catheters are meticulously prevented from moving during patient transport. Most series describe excellent safety and low morbidity, but occasional technique-related complications have contributed to controversy regarding this procedure. Vascular complications, such as popliteal artery thrombosis and iliac artery thrombosis, were initially reported by Sewell et al. (2006) and Greenberg et al. (2007) [1, 2]. Similar cases of arterial complication were subsequently reported by other authors.

References

1. Sewell MF, Rosenblum D, Ehrenberg H. Arterial embolus during common iliac balloon catheterization at cesarean hysterectomy. Obstet Gynecol. 2006;108:746–8.
2. Greenberg JI, Suliman A, Iranpour P, et al. Prophylactic balloon occlusion of the internal iliac arteries to treat abnormal placentation: a cautionary case. Am J Obstet Gynecol. 2007;197(5):470e1–4.

Application and Methods of Arterial Embolization for Prophylaxis and Treatment of Massive Hemorrhage in Obstetric Fields

3

Shinsuke Kyogoku

Abstract
Large volumes of obstetric bleeding are often transferred to DIC and the mortality rate is high. In the obstetric field, diseases causing massive bleeding that can be lethal include those from cervical pregnancy in early pregnancy to postpartum bleeding, and the ones responded by hysterectomy. In the recent years it has become possible to preserve the uterus by controlling bleeding by the development of interventional radiology (IVR).In this chapter, we list the diseases and conditions subject to IVR and explain about selection and manipulation of "catheter of arterial embolization" and embolic material; outlines of prophylactic and emergency adaptation of "balloon occlusion," and "postoperative grades" and "complications" are also outlined.

Keywords
Obstetrical hemorrhage · IVR (interventional radiology) · Arterial embolization
Balloon occlusion

3.1 Introduction

Massive obstetrical hemorrhage often arises when impaired coagulation caused by fibrinogen depletion resulting from amniotic fluid embolism evolves into DIC and carries a high mortality rate. In the field of obstetrics, conditions that can lead to fatal massive hemorrhage include cervical pregnancy of the first trimester and postpartum hemorrhage (Table 3.1). Such massive hemorrhage had formerly been treated by

S. Kyogoku
Department of Radiology, Juntendo Urayasu Hospital, Urayasu, Japan
e-mail: skyogoku@juntendo-urayasu.jp

S. Takeda, R. Kuwatsuru (eds.), *Gynecologic and Obstetric Prophylactic Hemostasis by Intra-arterial Balloon Occlusion*, https://doi.org/10.1007/978-981-10-8833-9_3

Table 3.1 Obstetric hemorrhagic condition

Prepartum
Extra uterine (ectopic) pregnancy
Fallopian tube pregnancy, ovarian pregnancy, abdominal pregnancy
Cervical pregnancy
Cesarean scar pregnancy
Placental abruption
Placenta previa, placenta accrete
Uterine rupture
Postpartum
Atonic hemorrhage
Uterine inversion
Birth canal damage
Vaginal laceration, perineal laceration, uterine rupture
Retained placenta (placental polyp)

hysterectomy; however, with the development of interventional radiology (IVR), the hemorrhage can now be controlled while maintaining fertility by preserving the uterus. Treatment methods for obstetrical hemorrhage include administration of uterotonics, bimanual compression of the uterus, uterine gauze filling, and balloon tamponade. When hemostasis is not achieved despite such attempts, then IVR is performed [1–3].

Diseases and conditions subject to IVR include cervical pregnancy, Cesarean scar pregnancy, placenta previa, and placenta accreta during pregnancy. During intrapartum and at birth, atonic hemorrhage (uterine contractile dysfunction), birth canal damage (vaginal laceration and perineal laceration), uterine rupture, residual placental fragments, and placental polyp can occur. In most of these conditions, arterial embolization of the responsible artery such as the internal iliac artery, the uterine artery, and the internal pudendal artery is performed. In the event of placenta previa and placenta accreta, delivery by Cesarean section is selected. However, if placental abruption occurs, it causes massive hemorrhage; therefore, an occlusion balloon is placed in one of the arteries among the bilateral common iliac arteries, internal iliac artery, or abdominal aorta prior to surgery to control blood flow in the event of hemorrhage (preventive IVR). In case that placental separation did not occur and hemorrhage was avoided, hysterectomy may be performed after the fetus is delivered. In such case, combination of balloon occlusion of the artery and arterial embolization is performed.

3.2 Preoperative Evaluation

Prior to IVR treatment, the patient's underlying diseases, clinical course, and background should be reviewed. It is also important to ascertain the patient's general condition. However, it is difficult to accurately determine the amount of blood loss at delivery because it is intermixed with amniotic fluid. Therefore, it is important to evaluate using the shock index (Table 3.2) or the obstetric disseminated intravascular coagulation (DIC) score (Table 3.3) [4]. When shock index ≥ 1.5, obstetric DIC

Table 3.2 Shock index (SI)

SI = heart rate/systolic blood pressure
→ SI = 1 means 1,500 cc blood loss, SI = 1.5 means 2,500 cc blood loss

Table 3.3 Obstetrical DIC score

Total score below ≥ 8, should be treat as 'obstetrical critical hemorrhage'		
1. Underlying diseases[a]	(choose one that apply)	(Score)
(a) Placental abruption		
• Stiffening of the uterus, death of the fetus		(5)
• Stiffening of the uterus, survival of the fetus		(4)
• Confirmatory diagnosis of placental abruption by ultrasonic tomographic findings and CTG findings		(4)
(b) Amniotic fluid embolism		
• Acute cor pulmonale		(4)
• Artificial ventilation		(3)
• Assisted respiration		(2)
• Oxygen flux alone		(1)
(c) DIC-type postpartum hemorrhage		
• In case the blood from the uterus has low coagulability		(4)
• Hemorrhage of 2000 mL ≤ (within 24 h after the start of hemorrhage)		(3)
• Hemorrhage of 1000 mL ≤, but not exceeding 2000 mL (within 24 h after the start of hemorrhage)		(1)
(d) Eclampsia		
• Eclamptic attack		(4)
(e) Severe infection		
• Those with fever accompanied by shock, bacteremia, and endotoxemia		(4)
• Continued fever or remittent fever		(1)
(f) Other underlying diseases		(1)
2. Clinical symptoms		
(a) Acute renal failure	(choose one that apply)	
• Anuria (≤5 mL/h)		(4)
• Oliguria (5–20 mL/h)		(3)
(b) Acute respiratory failure (amniotic fluid embolism excluded)	(choose one that apply)	
• Artificial ventilation or occasional assisted respiration		(4)
• Oxygen flux alone		(1)
(c) Organ failure	(choose all that apply)	
• Heart (rales or foamy sputum, etc.)		(4)
• Liver (visible jaundice, etc.)		(4)
• Brain (clouding of consciousness, convulsion, etc.)		(4)
• Digestive tract (necrotic enteritis, etc.)		(4)
• Other severe organ failure		(4)

(continued)

Table 3.3 (continued)

(d) Hemorrhage diathesis		(4)
Macroscopic hematuria and melena, purpura, hemorrhage from the mucous membrane, gingival bleeding, bleeding at the site of injection, etc.		
(e) Shock symptoms	(choose all that apply)	
• Pulse rate ≥100/min		(1)
• Blood pressure ≤90 mmHg (systolic) or blood pressure reduction of ≥40%		(1)
• Cold sweat		(1)
• Pallor		(1)
3. Laboratory findings	(choose all that apply)	
• Serum FDP ≥ 10 μg/mL		(1)
• Platelet counts ≤10 × 10^4/μL		(1)
• Fibrinogen ≤ 150 mg/dL		(1)
• PT ≥ 15 (s) (≤50%) or hepaplastin test ≤50%		(1)
• Erythrocyte sedimentation rate ≤ 4 mm/15 min or ≤15 mm/h		(1)
• Bleeding time ≥5 min		(1)
• Other coagulation and fibrinolysis factors; AT ≤ 18 mg/dL or ≤60%, prekallikrein, α2-Pl, plasminogen, other coagulation factors ≤50%		(1)

α2-pl α2-plasmin inhibitor, *AT* antithrombin, *CTG* cardiotocography, *DIC* disseminated intravascular coagulation, *FDP* fibrin degradation product, *PT* prothrombin time
[a]Only one of these items will be adopted as the score of underlying diseases

score ≥ 8 points, or abnormality in vital signs are observed, it is diagnosed as "obstetrical critical hemorrhage," and treatment including transfusion should be preceded immediately.

When performing IVR, it is recommended to perform non-contrast and contrast-enhanced (arterial and delayed phase) computed tomography (CT) before IVR (Fig. 3.1). In non-contrast CT, the presence or absence of hematoma and hemorrhagic ascites is investigated. In arterial phase contrast-enhanced CT, the presence or absence of pseudoaneurysm and slight blood vessel leakage are verified. When contrast medium diffusion is observed in the delayed phase, the causative lesion can be identified. Multiplanar reconstruction (MPR) allows images to be created in the coronal or sagittal plan, and if 3D VR (3D volume rendering) images of blood vessels are available, it can be useful for contrast-enhanced angiography (Figs. 3.2 and 3.3). In case of atonic hemorrhage following Cesarean section, the uterine artery is often the responsible vessel. In the event of hemorrhage following vaginal delivery, concurrent birth canal injury can be suspected, and the internal pudendal artery and the vaginal wall artery may be a responsible vessel. These facts are points to keep in mind for both CT and angiography, and image analysis should be performed while taking into account the delivery method such as Cesarean section or vaginal delivery.

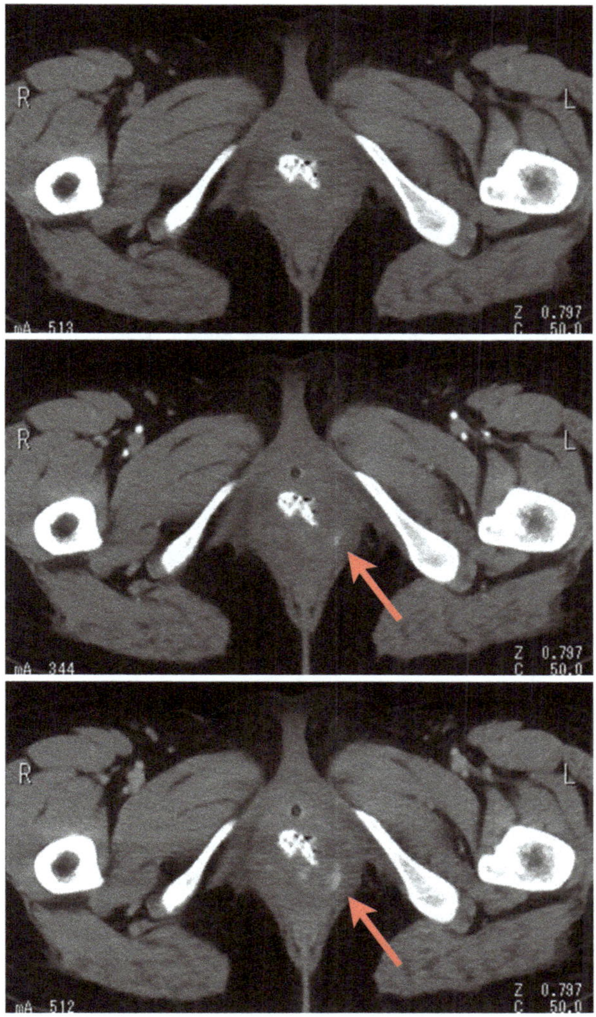

Fig. 3.1 A case of vaginal laceration: contrast enhanced CT (arterial phase) shows small enhanced spot in vaginal wall and spread at venous phase (arrow)

3.3 Transcatheter Arterial Embolization

In case of atonic hemorrhage following Cesarean section, particularly when emergency hemostasis is needed, bilateral uterine artery angiography and embolization should be performed. The femoral artery in the inguinal region is recommended as the puncture site as per normal angiography, and 4 Fr or 5 Fr short sheath (approximately 10 cm) is placed.

When identifying the hemorrhage site, aortic angiography using a pigtail catheter (Fig. 3.4) is recommended, and the catheter tip needs to be placed at the renal artery level upstream of the origin of the ovarian artery, in order to confirm the

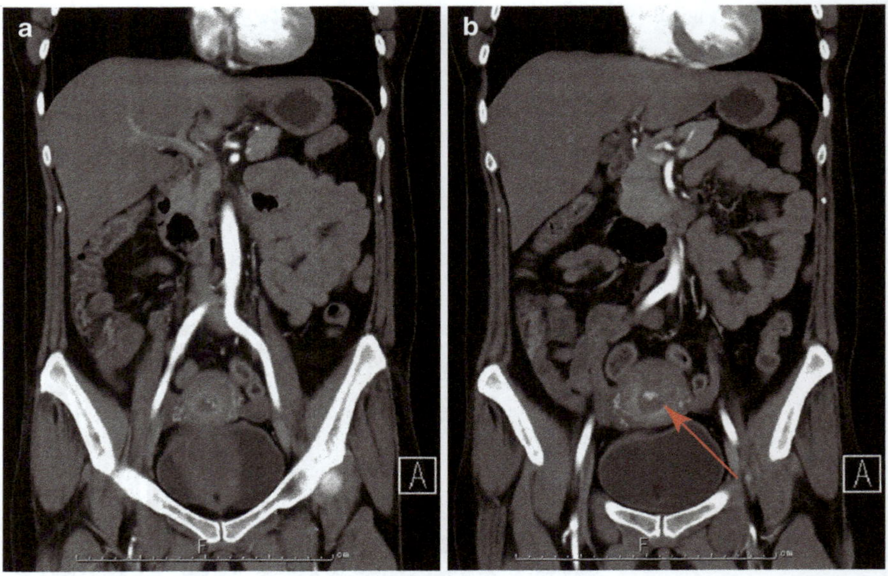

Fig. 3.2 (**a**) Multiplanar reconstruction (MPR); coronal or sagittal plane image made by MPR also provides helpful information for angiography

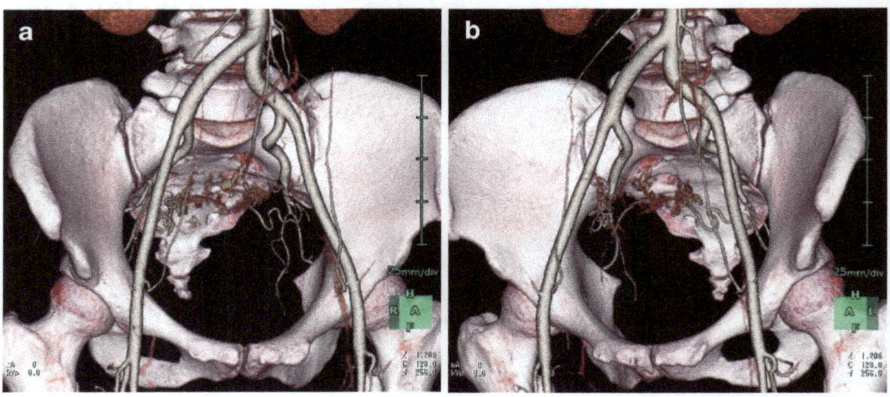

Fig. 3.3 (**a**, **b**) 3D volume rendering (3DVR) image by creating and rotating a 3D image; identification of the beginning of uterine artery is facilitated

involvement of the ovarian artery. However, this procedure may be omitted if the patient's condition is unstable and there is little time.

When the responsible vessel and hemorrhage point can be confirmed by leakage of contrast medium or pseudoaneurysm, selective embolization is preferable where possible. The catheter is advanced toward the hemorrhage site, and embolization is performed using a gelatin sponge, N-butyl cyanoacrylate (NBCA), or a metallic

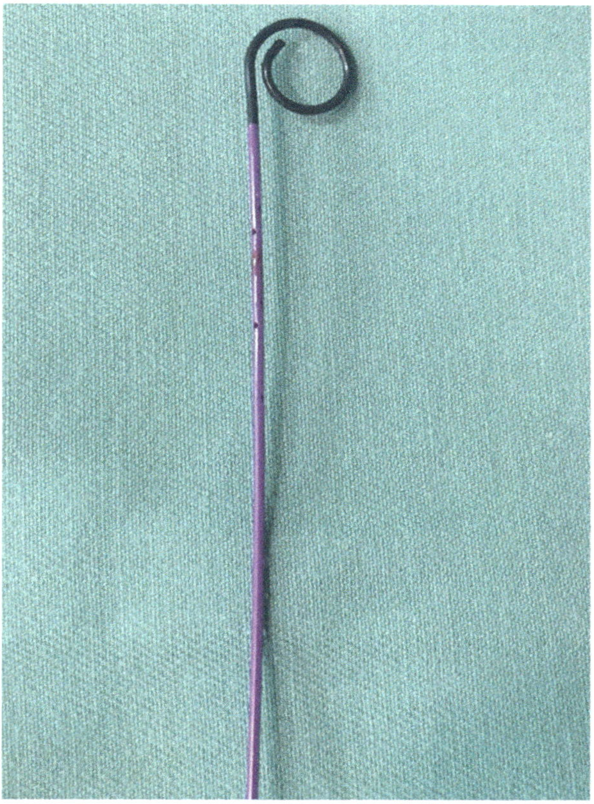

Fig. 3.4 Pigtail catheter: coiled catheter like "pigtail" with multiple side holes

embolization coil. In case of pseudoaneurysms, embolization is performed distal and proximal to the site, and it is important to interrupt blood flow from collateral circulation. In the event of leakage from the uterine artery, contralateral anastomosis should be considered, and contralateral arterial selective embolization should be performed in addition to ipsilateral selective embolization.

When the site of hemorrhage is not clearly identified, selective embolization of the bilateral uterine arteries should be targeted where possible. When advancing the catheter to the uterine artery, a general cobra catheter (Fig. 3.5) or a hook catheter (Fig. 3.6) is commonly used as the guiding catheter; however, the Mohri's loop catheter designed specifically for the uterine artery is also useful (Fig. 3.7) [5]. When it is difficult to identify the origin of the uterine artery in the frontal view, contralateral anterior oblique contrast enhancement of the internal iliac artery is useful. In any case, when inserting the catheter deeply into the uterine artery, the use of a microcatheter is recommended. In the event of accompanying laceration at birth following vaginal delivery, embolization including the vaginal branch of the uterine artery at the cervix is needed. However, when selective embolization of the uterine artery is difficult or when hemostasis cannot be achieved by embolization of the bilateral uterine arteries, then the internal pudendal artery, the obturator artery, or

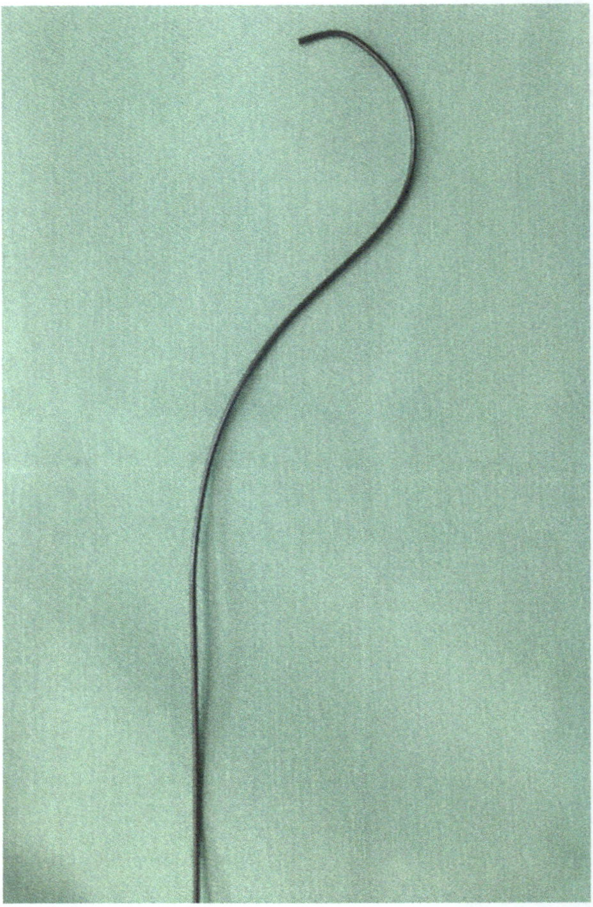

Fig. 3.5 Cobra catheter: shaped catheter like "cobra head"

the vaginal artery may be the site of hemorrhage. In such case, arterial embolization accessing from the anterior branch of the bilateral internal iliac arteries can be performed. However, when hemostasis is not achieved despite embolization of the anterior branches of the bilateral iliac arteries, hemorrhage from the ovarian artery, inferior epigastric artery, or external iliac artery is suspected. Therefore, the range of imaging should be expanded to identify the responsible artery for treatment (Figs. 3.8 and 3.9).

A gelatin sponge is generally used for the embolic material, and the method includes cutting with a scalpel or scissors or pumping with a syringe and stopcock. The latter method produces smaller particles and increases the risk of uterine necrosis, and thus caution is required to minimize the number of pumping. Other embolic materials include NBCA and metal embolization coils, which are permanent

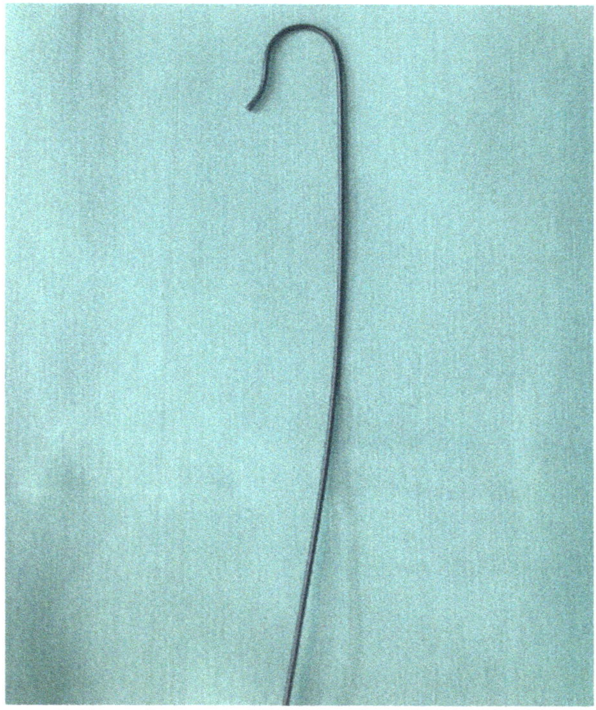

Fig. 3.6 Hook catheter: J-shaped catheter most commonly used

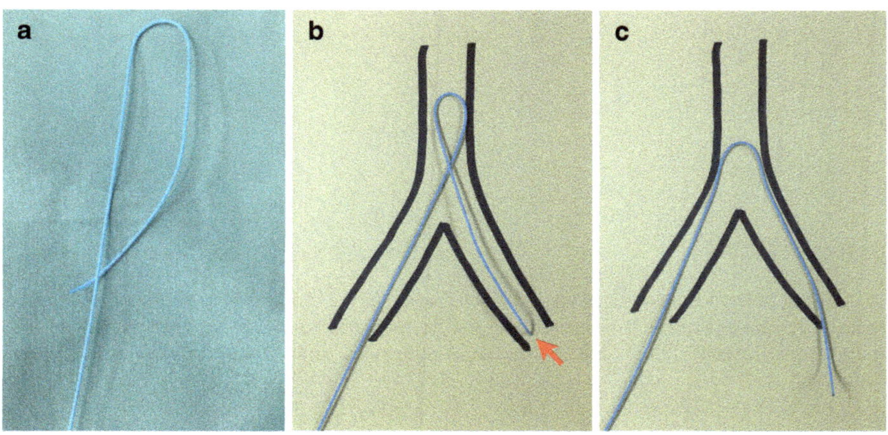

Fig. 3.7 (**a**) MOHRI type loop catheter: 3D-shaped catheter designed for uterine artery. In this figure, catheter tip is facing forward. (**b**) Making the loop makes the tip of the catheter face backward. In this figure, catheter tip is facing backward (arrow). This facilitates insertion into the internal iliac artery. (**c**) Thereafter, when the loop is released, catheter tip is turned forward again, and insertion into the uterine artery becomes easy

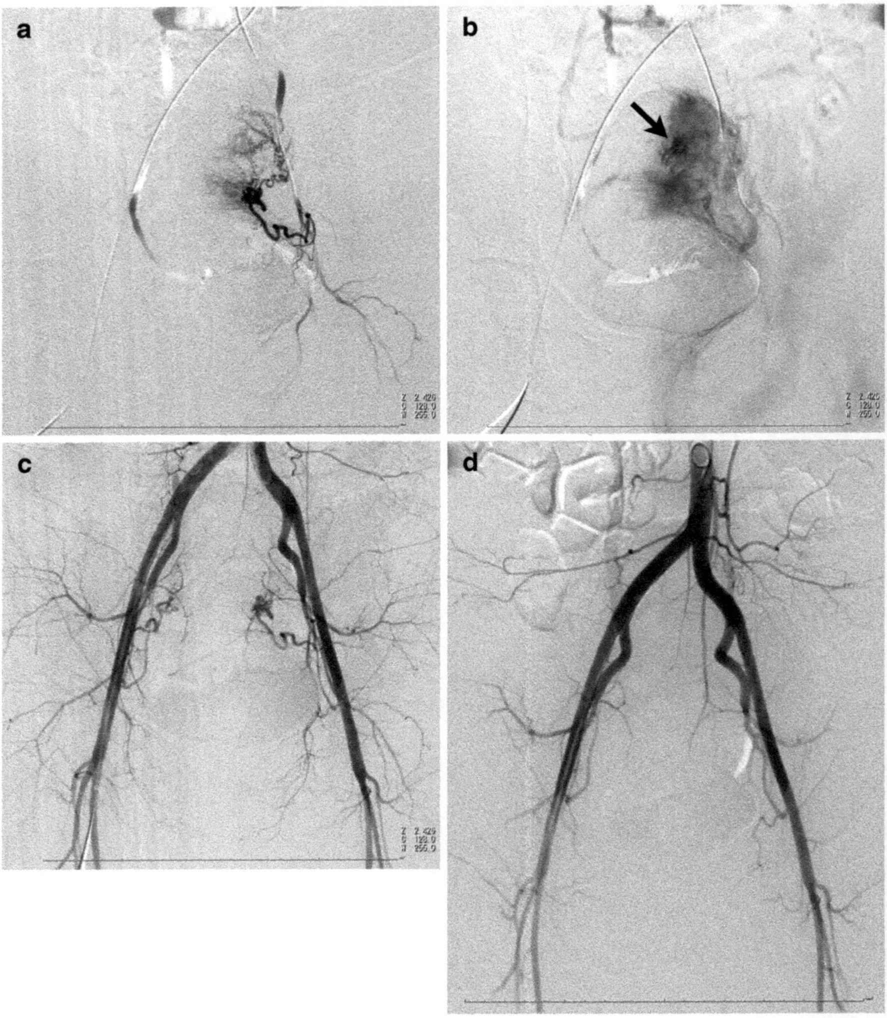

Fig. 3.8 (**a**) Selective angiography of Lt. uterine artery shows characteristic tortuous vessels. (**b**) In late phase, pooling of contrast medium suggesting uterine bleeding (arrow). (**c**) Bilateral uterine arterial embolization (UAE) was done. (**d**) Angiography after UAE, tortuous vessels are diminished

embolization materials, unlike gelatin sponge. NBCA demonstrates immediate effect and is expected to be effective in patients with low coagulability; however, it is difficult to manage and requires particular skill. The appropriate selection and combination of such materials should be investigated based on the characteristics of each material.

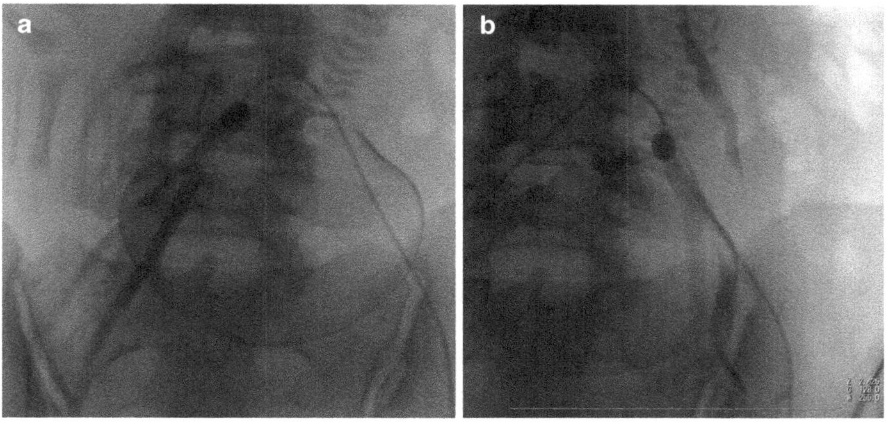

Fig. 3.9 (**a**, **b**) Occlusion balloon catheters were inserted bilaterally, positioned at common or internal iliac arteries. During placenta removal, inflate balloon to decrease bleeding

3.4 Artery Blockage with Balloon Catheter

3.4.1 Preventive Blockage with Balloon Catheter

In case of placenta previa and placenta accreta, massive hemorrhage is expected upon Cesarean section. When such conditions are suspected, preventive bleeding control can be attempted by balloon catheter placement. In that case, on the same day prior to a scheduled Cesarean section, bilateral inguinal punctures and insertion of balloon catheters into the bilateral common iliac arteries or bilateral internal iliac arteries are performed. The balloons are then inflated after delivery of the fetus to interrupt blood flow, thereby reducing the volume of blood loss. In general, a catheter with balloon with maximum diameter of approximately 10 mm and a sheath matched to the catheter are used to interrupt the internal iliac artery or the common iliac artery. The balloon catheter placement is performed on the contralateral side to the puncture site, passing across the aortic bifurcation and placing antegradely. When inflating the balloon, it is recommended to determine the catheter placement site taking into account that the site of occlusion may move slightly toward distal side due to blood flow.

3.4.2 Emergency Artery Blockage with Balloon Catheter

Emergency artery blockage with balloon catheter is performed as an urgent treatment for patients with deteriorated hemodynamics requiring prompt action. The blockage site is selected from the bilateral internal iliac arteries, the common iliac arteries, or the abdominal aorta. When the balloon catheter is placed in the aorta, it is preferable to select the site immediately beneath the renal artery bifurcation, in order to maintain renal blood flow. This is a temporary procedure to gain time until arterial embolization or surgical hemostasis can be performed. The instruments used for this procedure are in accordance with the preventive blockage procedure with balloon catheter; however, a balloon catheter with maximum diameter of approximately 30 mm is used for the aorta.

3.5 Postoperative Outcome and Complications

The clinical success of arterial embolization (IVR for acute hemorrhage) for postpartum hemorrhage is defined as "when there are no other surgical procedures required to achieve hemostasis," and the success rate has been reported to be approximately 90%. It has been reported that 8% of patients with obstetric massive hemorrhage undergo hysterectomy. The success rate of arterial embolization varies depending on the causes of postpartum hemorrhage, with the highest success rate observed for atonic hemorrhage, whereas the lower rate is noted for laceration of the birth canal and hemorrhagic shock [6].

The incidence of complications of IVR is 6–7%. The complications include general events associated with angiography such as inguinal hematoma and post-embolization syndrome, uterine necrosis associated with the embolization of target artery, intrauterine synechia (Asherman's syndrome), pelvic infection, amenorrhea, oligomenorrhea, bladder necrosis, buttock necrosis, and buttock claudication. Uterine necrosis is thought to occur more frequently when minute embolization materials are used. However, cases of uterine necrosis associated with gelatin sponge fragments have also been reported; thus, countermeasures such as reducing the number of pumping should be considered. There have been no reports of fatal case caused by complications, and reported fatal cases have been thought to occur due to intracerebral hemorrhage or hemorrhage associated with coagulopathy.

Conclusion

With the rise in awareness of IVR and increased recognition of its efficacy, obstetricians have growing expectations for radiologists (IVR specialists). Consequently, the frequency of hysterectomy performed for hemorrhage control has been on a decreasing trend. As the patients for indication are relatively young with minimal arteriosclerotic changes, IVR can be performed relatively easily if the procedure is performed promptly and reliably by a specialist with expertise in anatomical structures of pelvic vessels and properties of materials used for embolization.

References

1. Sentilhes L. Postpartum hemorrhage: guidelines for clinical practice from the French College of Gynaecologists and Obstetricians (CNGOF): in collaboration with the French Society of Anesthesiology and Intensive Care (SFAR). Eur J Obstet Gynecol Reprod Biol. 2015;198:12–21.
2. Nohira T, Onodera T, Isaka K. Emergency postpartum hysterectomy: incidence, trends, indications, and complications. Hypertens Res Pregnancy. 2014;2(2):88–93.
3. Farsad K. Postpartum pelvic hemorrhage. In: Jean-Francois HG, editor. Abrams' angiography: interventional radiology. Philadelphia: Lippincott Williams & Wilkins; 2013. p. 291–7.
4. Kobayashi T. Obstetrical disseminated intravascular coagulation score. J Obstet Gynecol Res. 2014;40:1500–6.
5. Mohri M. Simplified bilateral selective catheterization of the uterine artery. Radiology. 1978;129:239–41.
6. Ruiz Labarta FJ. Outcomes of pelvic arterial embolization in the management of postpartum hemorrhage: a case series study and systematic review. Eur J Obstet Gynecol Reprod Biol. 2016;206:12–21.

4 Temporary Endovascular Balloon Occlusion of the Internal Iliac Arteries to Prevent Hemorrhage During Uterine Cervical Myomectomy

Tsuyoshi Ota and Hiroshi Kaneda

Abstract

Cervical myomectomy carries a significant risk of hemorrhagic complications. Herein, we describe a prophylactic procedure—temporary endovascular balloon occlusion of the internal iliac arteries—that can be used to prevent excessive bleeding during surgical removal of a huge uterine cervical myoma. Endovascular occlusion catheters are placed in both internal iliac arteries. During myomectomy, the balloons are inflated to occlude these vessels. Upon completion of the surgery, and thus after the myometrium is sutured, the balloons are deflated, hemostasis is confirmed, and the catheters are removed. Thus far, we have used this method to reduce blood loss in 16 patients undergoing cervical myomectomy, and there has been no adverse effect. We have found the procedure, which we describe in detail, to be useful not only for the patients undergoing simple cervical myomectomy but also for the patients requiring cervical myomectomy concomitant with hysterectomy.

Keywords

Uterine cervical myoma · Endovascular balloon occlusion · Hemorrhage

T. Ota
Department of Obstetrics and Gynaecology, Faculty of Medicine, Juntendo University, Tokyo, Japan
e-mail: tota@juntendo.ac.jp

H. Kaneda (✉)
Department of Obstetrics and Gynaecology, Faculty of Medicine, Juntendo University, Tokyo, Japan

Department of Obstetrics and Gynaecology, Shizuoka Hospital, Juntendo University, Izunokuni, Shizuoka, Japan
e-mail: hrs-knd@juntendo.ac.jp

S. Takeda, R. Kuwatsuru (eds.), *Gynecologic and Obstetric Prophylactic Hemostasis by Intra-arterial Balloon Occlusion*, https://doi.org/10.1007/978-981-10-8833-9_4

4.1 Introduction

Leiomyomas is the most common uterine neoplasm in women of reproductive age [1]. Hysterectomy is a definitive solution, but many young women with a leiomyoma wish to preserve their fertility and desire more conservative surgical therapy. Uterine cervical myoma accounts for fewer than 5% and of all leiomyomas, but cervical myomectomy poses a significant risk of hemorrhagic complications [2]. Blood supply to the cervical myoma derives from the descending branch of the uterine artery and the vaginal artery, both of which originate from the internal iliac artery. Several methods aimed at decreasing blood loss during myomectomy have been introduced, including preoperative GnRH agonist therapy [3]; tourniquet application, as described by Bonney or Rubin [4]; intraoperative myometrial injection of vasopressin [5]; and temporary clamping of the uterine artery or internal iliac artery [3]. Here we describe temporary endovascular balloon occlusion of both internal iliac arteries, a method we have used recently to reduce blood loss in patients undergoing surgical removal of huge cervical myoma. The method was first described as a means of controlling bleeding during cesarean section or cesarean hysterectomy in patients with a placental implantation disorder such as placenta previa or placenta increta [6].

4.2 Methods

4.2.1 Indication and Preparation

Temporary endovascular balloon occlusion is applicable to patients undergoing surgical removal of a uterine cervical myoma node that is over 10 cm or that results in hypermenorrhea or sterility. In addition to the abnormally frequent or heavy menstruation, the hypermenorrhea may be characterized by frequent urination. Magnetic resonance imaging (MRI) is performed to assess and precisely localize the myoma node. Generally, the node distorts the cervix anatomically, making MRI localization necessary. Computed tomographic angiography is performed to identify the vascular distribution of the myoma and the uterus. Images of representative cervical myomas for which the procedure is applicable are shown in Fig. 4.1. Upon confirmation of the cervical myoma, gonadotropin-releasing hormone (GnRH) agonist is injected every 4 weeks for 3–6 months to shrink the myoma and migrate the anemia, if present. Autologous blood is collected by a blood transfusion service 1–3 weeks before the planned surgery. If the myoma is located on the posterior wall of the cervix, bilateral ureteral stenting is considered to prevent ureteral injury, and in such cases, the stents are usually inserted by a urologist in advance of the fibroid removal surgery. The stenting allows for easy identification of the ureters during the surgery.

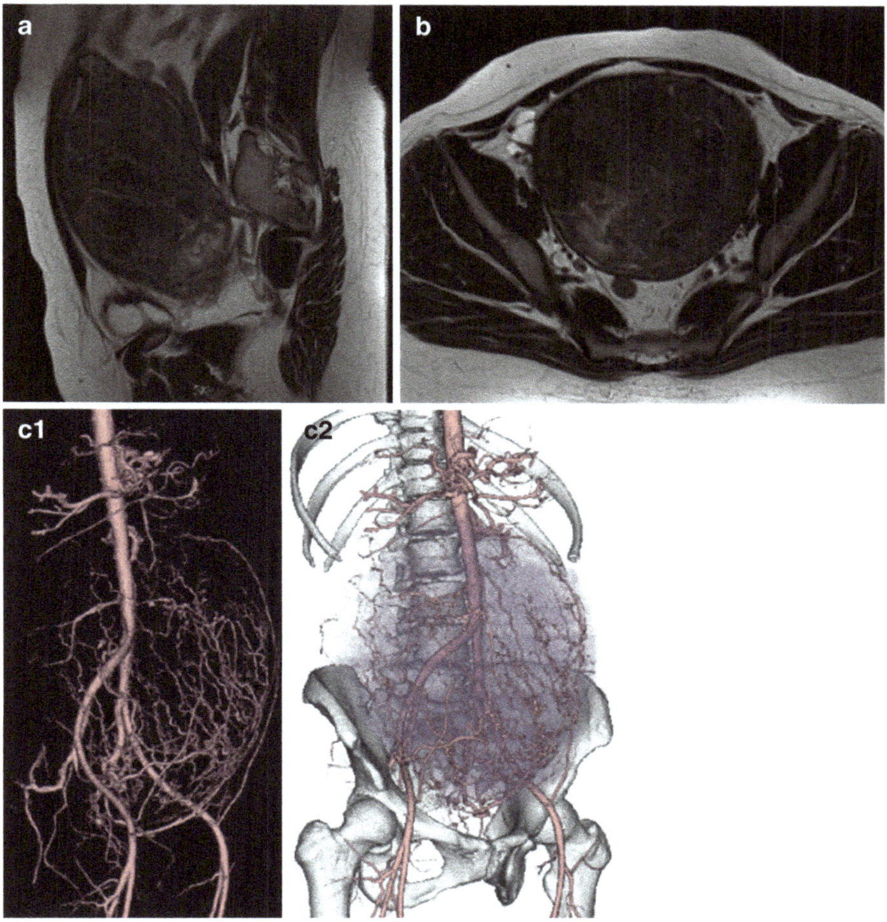

Fig. 4.1 Images of uterine cervical myomas for which the temporary endovascular balloon occlusion procedure was effective in preventing excessive blood loss during myomectomy (**a**) Magnetic resonance (MR) T2-weighted sagittal image of a myoma located on the posterior uterine cervical wall. The myoma is 25 cm in diameter. The endometrium of the uterine body is clearly visualized, and the cervical canal appears elongated. (**b**) MR T2-weighted axial image of a huge cervical myoma occupying the pelvic cavity. In such cases, the huge myoma node makes ligation of the internal iliac artery and uterine artery difficult. (**c**, 1 and 2) Reconstructed preoperative computed tomography angiogram of cervical myoma and surrounding vessels shows prominent vascularization originating from the uterine artery

4.2.2 Insertion of the Balloon Catheters

The occlusion catheters are inserted just before surgery. This is done in the angiography suite, where an interventional radiologist inserts balloon catheters into the iliac arteries via the femoral arteries (see Chap. 2 for detailed description of the catheterization procedure).

4.2.3 Surgical Procedure

Once the patient is transported to the operating room, pulse oximeters are placed, one on the patient's right big toe and the other on the left big toe, so that arterial oxygen saturation can be monitored throughout the surgery.

The iliac arteries were then temporarily occluded by inflation of the catheter balloons, and a dilute solution of vasopressin (X-100) is injected into the myometrium around the myoma node. A horizontal incision is made in the uterus, and myoma screw node is used to remove the fibroid. After its removal, multiple Z-sutures are placed in the myoma bed to ensure hemostasis, and the bed is carefully closed with two or three layers of sutures to avoid the creation of any dead space. After complete hemostasis is completed, the catheter balloons are deflated, and the myomectomy site is carefully inspected. A drain is placed in the pelvic cavity, and the balloon catheters are removed. This completes the operation. The drain is removed the next day, once hemostasis is reconfirmed.

It is important to note that the balloon occlusion time should not exceed 60 min to avoid lower extremity peripheral neuropathy, pudendal nerve paralysis, and complications from ischemia such as tissue necrosis. It is important to monitor the oxygen saturation of the blood flow from the external iliac artery to the femoral artery with a pulse oximeter at the periphery of the lower limb which had been done during surgery. If during the surgery it seemed that the occlusion time will exceed 60 min, the balloons should be deflated and then reinflated after 5 min.

When a patient with a huge cervical myoma is scheduled for hysterectomy, we sometimes remove the myoma nodule before the hysterectomy is initiated. The endovascular balloon occlusion procedure described above is useful for reducing blood loss in these patients.

4.3 Outcomes to Date

4.3.1 Operative Variables

To date, we have temporarily occluded both internal iliac arteries with the use of endovascular balloon catheters in 16 patients undergoing uterine cervical myomectomy. Clinical characteristics of the 16 patients are shown in Table 4.1. The patients ranged in age from 20 to 44 (mean, 34.9) years and were treated between October 2007 and April 2016. All underwent autologous blood donation preoperatively. GnRH agonist was injected three to six (mean, 4.4) times in each patient. Total operative time ranged from 53 to 308 (mean, 158.4) min, and the bilateral endovascular balloon occlusion time was 53.5 (25–77) min. The blood loss volume ranged from 30 to 1962 (mean, 637.9) μg, and none of the patients required blood transfusion. The excised specimens weighted 470–10,500 (mean, 2222) μg.

Table 4.1 Clinical characteristics of the patients who underwent myomectomy of huge uterine cervical myoma

Patient number	Old	Tumor diameter (cm)	Pre OP	Occlusion time (min)	Duration (min)	Blood loss (g)	Weight of specimen (g)	Autologus blood (mL)	Blood transfusion	Fertility results
1	31	40	GnRHa*5	35	183	505	10,500	500	(−)	
1	40	25	GnRHa*6	42	215	1220	1660	400	(−)	
3	40	25	GnRHa*3	60	129	520	1400	(−)	(−)	
4	28	25	GnRHa*6	63	206	1310	2460	800	(−)	Spontaneous abortion
5	34	20	GnRHa*2	60	192	380	1350	400	(−)	
6	37	25	GnRHa*5	60	218	1962	2715	400	(−)	
7	31	23	GnRHa*6	69	129	920	1700	400	(−)	Spontaneous abortion
8	37	19	GnRHa*5	60	127	735	1200	400	(−)	Normal delivery at 38 weeks
9	37	22	GnRHa*6	52	126	80	2000	400	(−)	
10	41	16	GnRHa*3	35	117	70	800	(−)	(−)	
11	20	11	GnRHa*5	77	196	580	470	(−)	(−)	
12	37	20	GnRHa*3	53	133	710	2900	400	(−)	
13	29	26	GnRHa*3	60	308	580	3300	(−)	(−)	
14	44	12	GnRHa*3	40	98	30	900	(−)	(−)	
15	40	24	GnRHa*4	65	104	225	1400	400	(−)	
16	33	12	GnRHa*6	25	53	380	800	(−)	(−)	

4.3.2 Operative and Immediate Postoperative Course

The operative and immediate postoperative course was without complications in all 15 cases.

4.3.3 Late Outcomes

Menstrual bleeding returned to normal after the surgery in all 15 patients, and none suffered cervical canal constriction.

4.3.4 Fertility Results

Three of the 16 patients conceived after myomectomy, but 2 of these 3 patients suffered a spontaneous abortion during. The third patient delivered a healthy baby at 38 gestational weeks, and there had been no sign of cervical incompetency and premature labor.

4.4 Case: Huge Uterine Cervical Myoma

A 28-year-old non-gravidity woman complained of abdominal bloating since 6 months. She had no history of irregular menstruation or dysmenorrhea, and there was nothing of note in her medical history and family history.

Physical examination showed no abnormality other than a large round abdomen and a swollen hard solid tumor in her abdomen. Blood tests showed mild anemia with a hemoglobin value of 10.0 g/dL. By vaginal examination the uterine cervix was difficult to identify owing to compression and distortion by huge cervical myoma. MRI showed a 25 cm fibroid in the anterior uterine cervix, and a normal uterine body was seen on top of the fibroid; the patient was diagnosed with a huge cervical fibroid (Fig. 4.1a, b). CT angiography was performed to identify the vascular distribution of the myoma and the uterus (Figs. 4.1c and 4.2).

Abdominal myomectomy was the surgical treatment selected, owing to the patient's hopes for further pregnancy. We carried out temporary endovascular balloon occlusion of both internal iliac arteries in order to reduce hemorrhage during cervical myomectomy for the huge cervical fibroid. Preoperative autologous blood donation was obtained by the blood transfusion service by drawing 400 mL of blood 2 weeks before surgery.

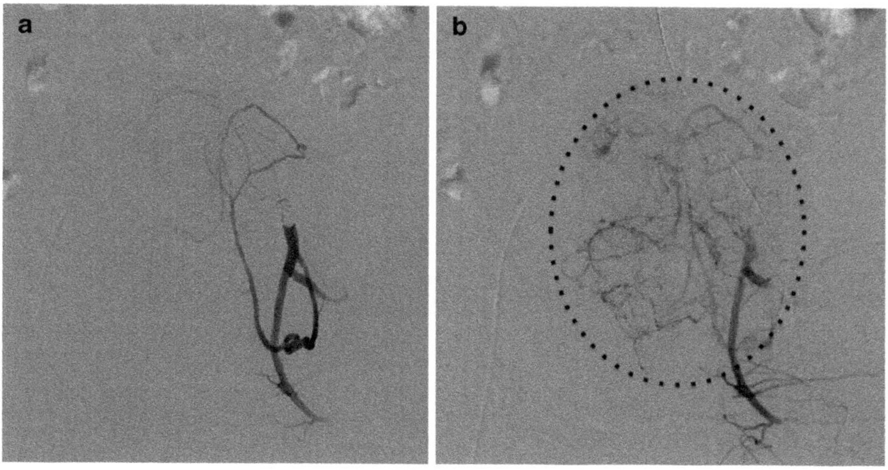

Fig. 4.2 Computed tomography angiograms obtained during insertion of the occlusion catheters (**a**) In this case, balloon occlusion of the left internal iliac artery was achieved by feeding the catheter through the right common femoral artery. Intravenous contrast injection while the balloon was inflated revealed stagnant flow. (**b**) In this case also, balloon occlusion of the left internal iliac artery was achieved by feeding the catheter through the right common femoral artery. Occlusion of the encircled vessels supplying blood to the cervical myoma and the uterus was confirmed during surgery

On the day prior to surgery, catheterization was performed with the assistance of an interventional radiologist, and we made sure of the blood flow to fibroid from mainly uterine arteries and blockade the flow by the balloon catheter (Fig. 4.2). In laparotomy, we were required to pay significant attention to the possibility of bladder injury because of the close proximity of the huge myoma. The position of the cervix had to be confirmed, and an incision was performed with care to avoid damage to the cervix (Fig. 4.3a). The uterine arteries were occluded by inflation of the balloon in the bilateral internal iliac artery and injection of vasopressin into the myometrium. Cervical myomectomy was performed with care so as not to injure arterioles and venous plexus around the cervical myoma and in the parametrium (Fig. 4.3b). Suturing was not carried out not to leave dead space after resection of the fibroid (Fig. 4.3c). After the removal site was sutured, we deflated the balloon, thus restoring blood flow to the pelvis and the uterus. After deflation, we made sure that there was no bleeding from the wound sites and then closed the abdominal wound. The total blood loss during the surgery was 505 ml, and the weight of specimen was 2460 g (Fig. 4.3d). There was no need for allogenic blood transfusion.

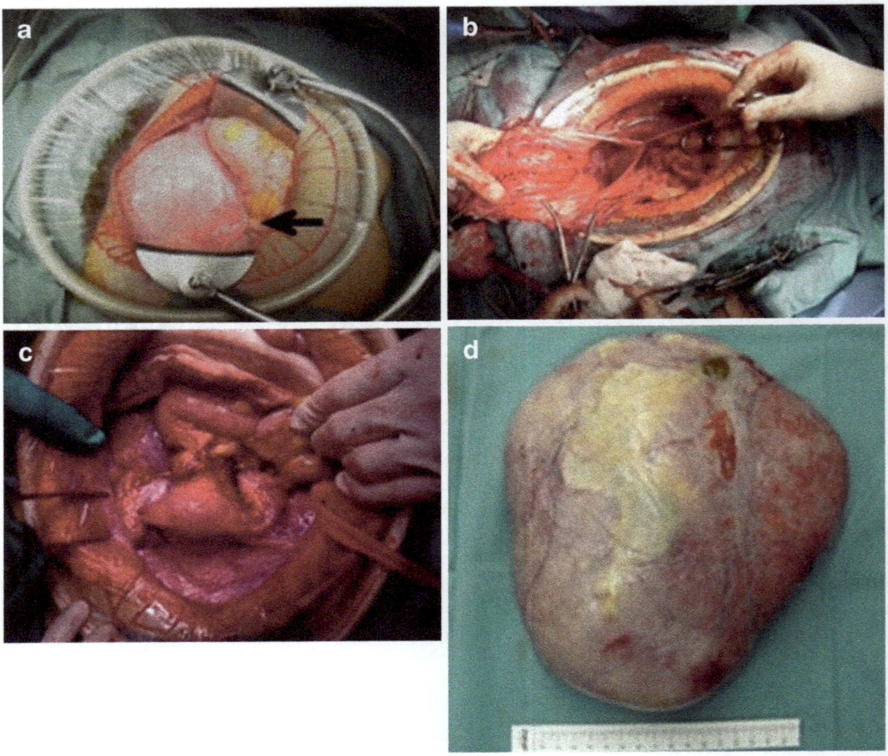

Fig. 4.3 Cervical myomectomy with occlusion catheters. (**a**) The position of the cervix confirmed under the normal uterine body (→) (**b**) Cervical myomectomy with care not to injure the cervix and the uterine arteriovenous. (**c**) After suturing the removal site not to leave dead space and deflation the balloon, there was no bleeding from the wound sites. (**d**) Total blood loss, 505 ml, and the weight of specimen, 2,460 g

Conclusion

We have introduced prophylactic procedure—temporary endovascular occlusion of both internal iliac arteries—to reduce the risk of hemorrhage in patients undergoing cervical myomectomy for a huge or symptomatic cervical myoma. Occlusion of the vessels that supply the cervical myoma was successful without any complications and blood transfusion. The method is useful not only for patients undergoing myomectomy but also for the patients undergoing hysterectomy for a huge cervical myoma. The procedure is easy to perform, it is safe, and transfusion can be avoided.

References

1. Solomon LA, Schimp VL, Ali-Fehmi R, et al. Clinical update of smooth muscle tumors of the uterus. J Minim Invasive Gynecol. 2005;12:401–8.
2. Chang WC, Chen SY, Huang SC, et al. Strategy of cervical myomectomy under laparotomy. Fertil Steril. 2010;94:2710–5.
3. Friedman AJ, Rein MS, Harrison-Atlas D, et al. A randomized, placebo-controlled, double-blind study evaluating leuprolide acetate depot treatment before myomectomy. Fertil Steril. 1989;52:728–33.
4. Rubin IC. The pericervical broad ligament tourniquet for preventive hemostasis in myomectomy. Obstet Gynecol. 1953;1:668–71.
5. Fletcher H, Frederick J, Hardie M, Simeon D. A randomized comparison of vasopressin and tourniquet as hemostatic agents during myomectomy. Obstet Gynecol. 1996;87:1014–8.
6. Dubois J, Garel L, Grignon A, et al. Placenta percreta: balloon occlusion and embolization of the internal iliac arteries to reduce intraoperative blood losses. Am J Obstet Gynecol. 1997;176:723–6.

Temporary Arterial Balloon Occlusion for Obstetrical Field

5

Jun Takeda and Shintaro Makino

Abstract

There are three main arteries for the balloon insertion: ventral aorta, common iliac arteries, and internal iliac arteries. In this chapter, characteristic features of temporary arterial balloon occlusion and strategies for the procedure are described.

Keywords

Hemorrhage · Placenta previa · Surgical technique · Temporary arterial balloon occlusion

5.1 Indication

There are two indications of the temporary intra-arterial balloon occlusion for massive obstetrics hemorrhage: prophylactic balloon occlusion and therapeutic balloon occlusion. The difference between the two procedures is the timing to apply sheath and balloon. Sheath and balloon are inserted before operation and inflated before the hemorrhagic procedure for the prophylactic balloon occlusion, while they are inserted and inflated during the hemorrhage for the therapeutic balloon occlusion. For the prophylactic balloon occlusion, placenta previa accreta, increta, and percreta are the good indications. To date, the indications expanded to the patient who

Electronic Supplementary Material The online version of this chapter (https://doi.org/10.1007/978-981-10-8833-9_5) contains supplementary material, which is available to authorized users.

J. Takeda (✉) · S. Makino
Department of Obstetrics and Gynecology,
Juntendo University Faculty of Medicine, Tokyo, Japan
e-mail: jtakeda@juntendo.ac.jp; shintaro@juntendo.ac.jp

S. Takeda, R. Kuwatsuru (eds.), *Gynecologic and Obstetric Prophylactic Hemostasis by Intra-arterial Balloon Occlusion*, https://doi.org/10.1007/978-981-10-8833-9_5

expected to have a massive bleeding because of myoma during cesarean section, because the patient with huge myoma tended to obtain myomectomy during cesarean section for avoiding lochiometra and infection and degeneration of the myoma. s for the therapeutic balloon occlusion, critical obstetric hemorrhage due to postpartum hemorrhage is the indication. The concept of resuscitative endovascular balloon occlusion of the aorta (REBOA) is also one of the topics recently. The procedure of the REBOA aims not only to stop bleeding but also reduce the blood stream for the lower half of the body and maintain cardiac preload and cerebral blood flow.

The strength of the prophylactic balloon occlusion is to allow the balloon inflation without vital sign instabilization. However, it is needed to be inserted during the pregnancy, thus the fetus exposed to radiation. In addition, prophylactic use of the balloon may include superfluous balloon insertions. No need to think about radiation exposure for the therapeutic balloon occlusion; however, the sheath and balloon needed to be inserted while massive bleeding with the vessel collapsed. Hence, obstetricians should carefully consider and choose whether to prophylactically insert the balloon or not.

5.2 Route

There are three main arteries for the balloon insertion (Fig. 5.1): ventral aorta (Video 5.1), common iliac arteries (Video 5.2), and internal iliac arteries (Video 5.3). Ventral aorta balloon occlusion or intra-aortic balloon occlusion was firstly

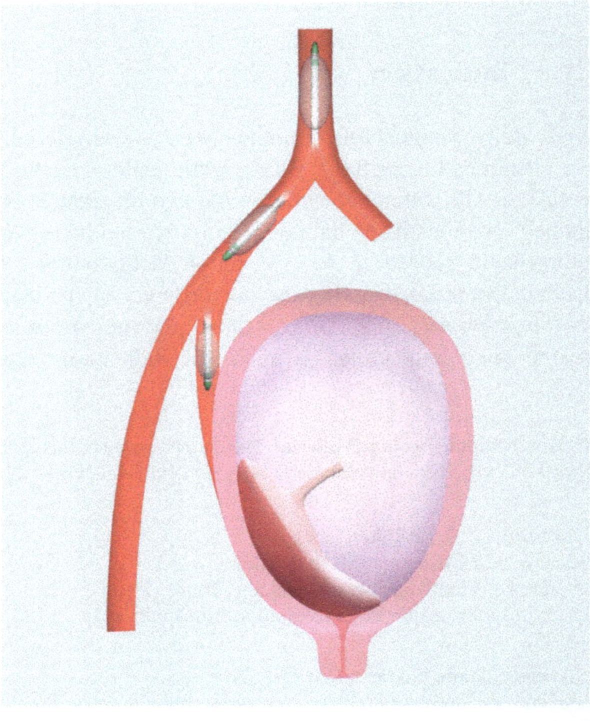

Fig. 5.1 The site of balloon occlusion. From top, intra-aortic balloon, common iliac balloon, and internal iliac balloon are shown

Table 5.1 The merit and demerit of each balloon occlusion

	Merit	Demerit
Intra-aortic balloon occlusion (IABO)	– High hemostatic effect – Single balloon insertion – Faster application – Allow for balloon insertion under ultrasonography	– Need for heparin administration and SpO2 monitoring in lower limbs – Not allowed for long balloon inflation
Internal iliac artery balloon occlusion (IIABO)	– Low incidence of ischemia for untargeted organs – No need for heparin administration and SpO2 monitoring in lower limbs	– Lower hemostatic effect because of regurgitant blood flow from the external iliac artery, especially in the case of placenta previa
Common iliac artery balloon occlusion (CIABO)	– Minimally invasive than IABO and superior effect than IIABO	– Need for heparin administration and SpO2 monitoring in lower limbs – Not allowed for long balloon inflation – Balloon displacement to the external iliac artery may cause rather massive bleeding

introduced 50 years ago for injured Korean War soldiers [1]. Conventionally, the balloon was inserted with cut down inguinal artery. Because of the complexity of artery cut down and in view of the risk of organ injury, smaller balloon to the peripheral artery becomes popular. However, internal iliac arteries are not able to decrease regurgitant blood flow from the external iliac artery via vaginal artery and other collateral arteries [2, 3]. Hence, common iliac artery balloon occlusion (CIABO) [4, 5] is now in common use. Obstetricians should inform those merits and demerits regarding balloon occlusion to the patient and family allow them to decide which surgical technique to adopt (Table 5.1).

5.3 Practical Aspects of the Procedure

Practical aspects of CIABO for placenta previa are described in this section. The algorism of the common iliac balloon occlusion during surgery is shown in Fig. 5.2.

1. Placement of the epidural anesthesia catheter

Placing the epidural anesthesia catheter in advance helps control pain at the time of inserting the common iliac artery balloon.

2. Placement of the occlusion balloon in the bilateral common iliac arteries

Performing magnetic resonance imaging before surgery in patients with suspected placenta previa accreta may provide the details and objective information of placenta.

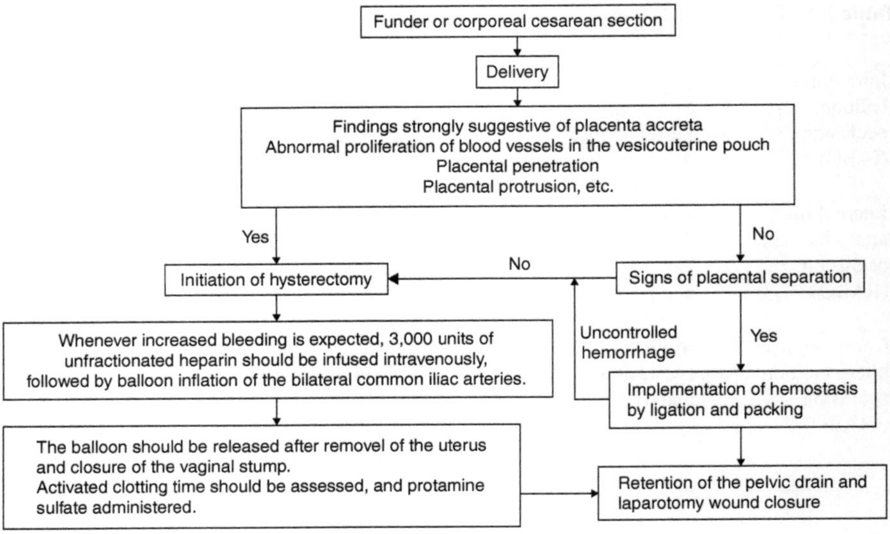

Fig. 5.2 The algorism of the common iliac balloon occlusion for placenta previa

The occlusion balloon inserted from the left inguinal region should be inserted in the right common iliac artery, whereas the one inserted from the right inguinal region should be inserted crosswise in the left common iliac artery. Test inflations of the balloons should, of necessity, be performed one at a time, and the fetal heart rate must be monitored continuously during these test inflations. If both balloons are inflated simultaneously during surgery, the balloons may become distended at a site more peripheral than expected. In particular, in cases with relatively short common iliac arteries, the balloon is more likely to enter the external iliac artery. Because of the nature of the catheter, it is apt to be displaced due to retrograde pressure. Therefore, it is important to retain the balloons crosswise in the artery contralateral to the insertion site to allow antegrade pressure to be exerted on the balloons. The exposure dose for catheter placement approached 70 mGy, at a maximum. The exposure dose to the fetus is considered to be lower and thus acceptable.

3. Confirmation of the surgical position, monitor, etc.

Because the sheath introducer is retained in the bilateral inguinal regions, bending of the hip joint may break the introducer. Thus, the surgical position should be broad base position.

In order to evaluate the efficacy of balloon occlusion and the influences on the lower limbs, a percutaneous oxygen saturation monitor (SpO2 monitor) is attached to both legs during surgery. Assuming massive bleeding, the arterial pressure line of the upper limb and the bilateral 18–14G venous lines are always secured.

4. Epidural anesthesia

It was difficult to achieve a sufficient bending position because the sheath introducer was retained in the bilateral inguinal regions. Thus, anesthesia should be given via epidural catheter which placed before the balloon insertion. It allows the mother to hear the initial birth cry of the neonate.

5. Initiation of cesarean section by abdominal longitudinal incision

A median incision large enough to ensure sufficient visualization is necessary for hysterectomy. A horizontal incision in the uterine fundus may help reducing bleeding amount. Therefore, it is not rare for us to extend the skin incision to a point above the navel.

6. Evaluation on necessity of the hysterectomy

After the cesarean section, the necessity of the hysterectomy should be evaluated with the laparotomy findings, bleeding amount, and vital signs.

7. Intravenous infusion of heparin

Administer intravenous infusion of heparin (e.g., 3000 units for unfractionated heparin) to prevent arterial thrombus prior to inflation of the balloon.

8. Inflation of the common iliac artery occlusion balloon

At the timing of hemorrhagic procedure, the balloons should be inflated one at a time. Balloon dilation should be limited to approximately 30 min to 1 h.

9. Confirmation of the attenuated internal iliac artery pulse and the attenuated SpO2 monitor waveforms in both lower limbs

To ensure that the balloon is properly inflated in the common iliac artery, attenuation of internal iliac artery pulse and waveforms from the SpO2 monitor in each leg should be confirmed. If the balloon enters the external iliac artery by error, continuation of the procedure raises the blood flow in the internal iliac artery and thereby further increases bleeding in the operative field, resulting in complete ischemia of the lower limbs.

There is no need for waveforms on the SpO2 monitor in each leg to disappear completely. Limited waveforms reflect a sufficient decrease in bleeding in the operative field. Conversely, if there is complete elimination of waveforms, it is necessary to confirm whether or not the balloon has entered the external iliac artery by error.

10. Deflation of the common iliac artery balloon occlusion

After the hemorrhagic procedure, the balloons should be deflated one at a time. If the blood flow in the lower limbs is completely blocked, the release of the balloon may lead to hyperkalemia. Therefore, attention should be paid to any changes in the T wave on the electrocardiographic monitor, and assessments of the potassium level in arterial blood gas analysis should be performed over time. In addition, attention should be paid to the acute changes of the blood pressure.

11. Administration of protamine sulfate

After release of the balloon, the activated clotting time (ACT) value should be determined, and if ACT is prolonged to more than 120 s, administration of protamine sulfate should be considered.

12. Search for the bleeding point, hemostasis, and closure of the wound

After the balloon deflation, rebleeding may occur. Therefore, it is necessary to add hemostatic procedure and drain tube insertion before the operative wound closure.

13. Removal of the balloon catheter and sheath introducer

The balloon catheters could be removed in the operating room after surgery. Consider removing the sheath introducer in the ward after confirming the absence of postoperative bleeding during and after the patient transfer, if necessary. Pressure at least 10 min of manual compression on the site of sheath introducer.

5.4 Case: Placenta Previa

A case which underwent cesarean hysterectomy due to placenta accreta employing CIABO.

The patient had previous cesarean section due to placenta previa and myoma. In the next pregnancy, placenta previa was recognized again. MRI (Fig. 5.3) and ultrasonography revealed that the uterine muscular layer was thin or defected without visible lacuna, thus placenta percreta was suspected. Elective cesarean was planned at 35 weeks of gestation. There was no request for the uterus preservation. On the operation day, CIABO was inserted by radiologists and she was moved to the operating room. Operation was started with the standby of the intraoperative blood salvage device. Placenta was existed just under the uterine serosa implicated placenta percreta. After the delivered of the neonate, hysterectomy was started, and CIABO was inflated just before bladder detachment after 3000 unit of heparin administration. After hysterectomy and hemostatic procedure, CIABO was deflated

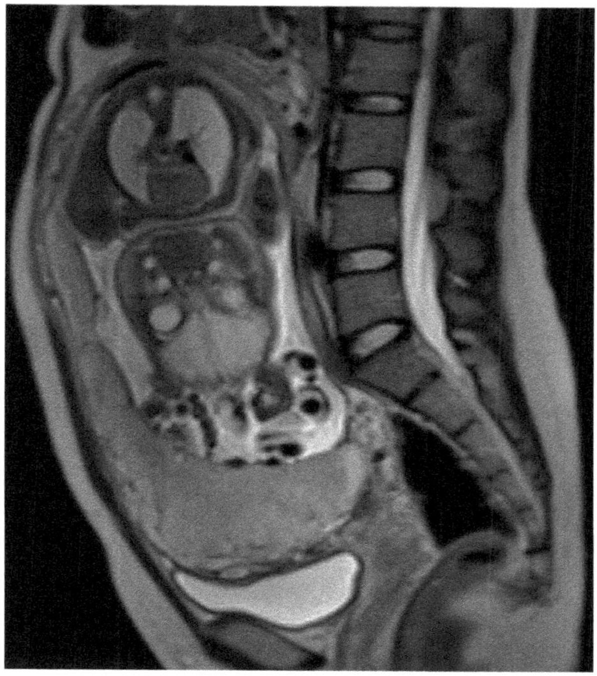

Fig. 5.3 MRI of placenta previa at 34 weeks of gestation. The uterine muscular layer was thin or defected at the placenta attachment site

one by one. Surgical duration was 130 min, and total blood loss was approximately 1800 mL; blood transfusion was not performed. The inflation time was 20 min. No remarkable complications exist, and she was discharged from the hospital 5 days after the surgery.

References

1. Hughes CW. Use of an intra-aortic balloon catheter tamponade for controlling intra-abdominal hemorrhage in man. Surgery. 1954;36:65–8.
2. Dubois J, Garel L, Grignon A, Lemay M, Leduc L. Placenta percreta: balloon occlusion and embolization of the internal iliac arteries to reduce intraoperative blood losses. Am J Obstet Gynecol. 1997;176(3):723–6.
3. Iwata A, Murayama Y, Itakura A, Baba K, Seki H, Takeda S. Limitations of internal iliac artery ligation for the reduction of intraoperative hemorrhage during cesarean hysterectomy in cases of placenta previa accreta. J Obstet Gynaecol Res. 2010;36(2):254–9. https://doi.org/10.1111/j.1447-0756.2009.01157.x.
4. Shih JC, Liu KL, Shyu MK. Temporary balloon occlusion of the common iliac artery: new approach to bleeding control during cesarean hysterectomy for placenta percreta. Am J Obstet Gynecol. 2005;193(5):1756–8.
5. Ono Y, Murayama Y, Era S, Matsunaga S, Nagai T, Osada H, Takai Y, Baba K, Takeda S, Seki H. Study of the utility and problems of common iliac artery balloon occlusion for placenta previa with accreta. J Obstet Gynaecol Res. 2018;44(3):456–62.

References

Lightning Source UK Ltd.
Milton Keynes UK
UKHW021132210319
339597UK00002B/12/P

9 789811 088322